Keto Diet (

This Keto Guide will take Care of your Time with Essential Recipes, and a special section for your Snack and Drink Keto.

by

TERRY ANDERSON

liable for any hardship or damages that may befall them after undertaking information described herein.

Additionally, the information in the following pages is intended only for informational purposes and should thus be thought of as universal. As befitting its nature, it is presented without assurance regarding its prolonged validity or interim quality. Trademarks that are mentioned are done without written consent and can in no way be considered an endorsement from the trademark holder.

Introduction

As women, when our age grows at 50, we are always looking for a quick and effective way to shed our excess weight, get our high blood sugar levels under control, reduce overall inflammation, and improve our physical and mental energy. It's frustrating to have all of these issues, especially the undeniable fats in our belly. Good thing that I found this great solution to all our worries when we reach this age level, and when our body gets weaker as time goes by. The ketogenic diet plans.

As a woman at this age, we all know that it is much more difficult for us to lose weight than men. I have lived on a starvation level diet and exercise like a triathlete and only lose five pounds. A man will stop putting dressing on his salad and will lose twenty pounds. It just not fair. But we have the fact that we are women to blame. Women naturally have more standing between themselves and weight loss than men do.

The mere fact that we, women, is the largest single contributor to why we find it difficult to lose weight. Since our bodies always think it needs to be prepared for a possible pregnancy, we will naturally have more body fat and less mass in our muscles than men.

Being in menopause will also cause us to add more pounds to our bodies, especially in the lower half. After menopause, our metabolism naturally slows down. Our hormone levels will decrease. These two factors alone will cause weight gain in the post-menopausal period.

There are numerous diet plan options offered to help shed weight, but the Ketogenic diet has been the most preferred lately. We've got many concerns around keto's effectiveness and exactly how to follow the diet plan in a healthy and balanced means.

The ketogenic diet for ladies at the age of over 50 is an easy and ideal way to shed extra pounds, stay energetic, and enjoy a healthy life. It balances hormones and improves our body capabilities without causing any harm to our overall wellness. Thus, if you are fighting post-menopausal symptoms and other health issues, you should do a keto diet right away!

A keto diet is a lifestyle, not a diet so, treat it like the same. The best way to approach keto to gain maximum benefits, especially for women over 50s, is to treat it as a lifestyle. You can't restrict your meal intake through obstructive and strict diets forever, right? It's the fundamental reason fad diets fail — we limit ourselves from too much to get rapid results, then we're are right back again at the weight where we started, or God forbid worse.

Keto is not a kind of diet that can be followed strictly forever — unless you need it as a therapeutic diet (i.e., epilepsy), a very narrow category. In the keto diet, we slowly transit into a curative state that we can withstand forever in a healthier way.

So, for me, being on a keto diet does not mean that I will be in ketosis forever. Instead, it means letting myself love consideration, such as a few desserts while vacationing or partying. It does not set me back to enjoy these desserts and let me consider it as the end of the diet. I can wake up the following morning and go back to the keto lifestyle, most suitable for me and my body consistently.

It allows my body to drastically boost its fat loss in many cases, decreasing pockets of undesirable fat.

With Keto Diet, it's not only giving weight loss assistance to reduce my weight, yet it can likewise ward off yearnings for unhealthy foods and protect me against Calories: collisions throughout the day. That is why I want to share with you how promising this Keto diet. As our age grow older, we must not let our body do the same. Focus your mindset on this fantastic diet, read, apply, and enjoy its best benefits.

What I promise you after you read the full guide of Keto Diet for Women after 50 and apply it to your daily lifestyle, especially the 30 days meal plan, you will achieve more than losing weight but also a new and improve healthier you!

CHAPTER 1: What Is the Ketogenic Diet?

he ketogenic diet is a perfect combination of an equal number of macros essential for the perfect and healthy functioning of the human body.

This diet is mostly focused on foods that are rich in fats, while carbohydrates are considerably lowered.

If you hadn't heard about the keto diet, you probably did not know that eating meals without balanced (or reduced) macros (carbohydrates, proteins, fats, and fibers) will lead to weight and fat.

When you provide your body with foods containing large amounts of carbohydrates (and fats and protein), your body stimulates insulin development, leading to leptin resistance. Slowly but surely, your body weight will increase. Not every organism is the same, but providing the b with unhealthy amounts of carbs combined with fats and proteins (without any physical activity) is a surefire way to end up obese.

How Was the Ketogenic Diet Discovered?

Although this diet may have only recently become popular, it is not new at all. It is almost a century old. In the early 1920s, Johns Hopkins Medical Center researchers had a mission to find a way to decrease the no. of seizures in epileptic children. It seemed like an impossible mission to help epileptic children. Still, after thorough research, the researchers discovered that food rich in carbohydrates is the main reason epileptic children have frequent seizures.

They decided to start a new diet and observe the results. The epileptic patients started following the ketogenic diet, which consisted of foods rich in fats and proteins. With only a small amount of carbohydrates, it was discovered that this diet significantly decreased the seizures.

However, as in everything, there were exceptions. The keto diet did not work for everyone; about 30 percent of epileptic children did not react to this diet.

Naturally, the epileptic children still had to be observed and take theirmedications, but the low-carb diet turned out to be quite a relief for most of them.

Before this research, some form of the keto diet had existed, even in ancient Greece and India. Fasting and reducing the consumption of foods with carbs was nothing new to these people. Historians have found ancient writings that carefully explained how a diet helps in managing epileptic seizures. In ancient times, people were giving up food for a day or two and were facing complete relief (especially people with epilepsy).

Because fasting can be quite a challenge, over time, the keto diet took on the form it has today. You get to eat enough, and you cut out only carbohydrates (or eat them in reduced amounts).

Before the Johns Hopkins Medical Center research, French doctors discovered a way to reduce epileptic seizures with suitable foods. At the beginning of the 20th century in France, an experiment was conducted in which about 20 patients with epilepsy followed a new diet (mostly vegetarian) that was low in carbs. By then, the doctors were using Potassium:

bromide to treat the patients, but it turned out that this did not work well in terms of their mental abilities. This early form of keto was combined with intermittent fasting and showed good results. About ten percent of the treated patients reacted positively to the new way of eating. Also, they were in a good mental state and did not need to take Potassium: bromide.

Slowly but surely, the ketogenic diet found its way to people without epilepsy. It was one of the diets that helped people stay full and healthy and lose weight fast.How Does the Keto Diet Work?

We will focus on how this diet works and how your body transitions from one way of functioning to another.

As mentioned before, the ketogenic diet was used mainly to lower the incidence of seizures in epileptic children. People wanted to check out how the keto diet would work with an entirely healthy person as things usually go.

This diet makes the body burn fats much faster than it does carbohydrates.

The carbohydrates that we take in through food are turned into glucose, one of the leading "brain foods." So, once you start following the keto diet, foods with reduced carbohydrates are forcing the liver to turn all the fats into fatty acids and ketone bodies. The ketones go to the brain and take the place of glucose, becoming the primary energy source.

This diet's primary purpose is to make your body switch from the way it used to function to an entirely new way of creating energy, keeping you healthy and alive.

Once you start following the ketogenic diet, you will notice that things are changing, first and foremost, in your mind. Before, carbohydrates were your main body 'fuel' and were used to create glucose so that your brain could function. Now you no longer feed yourself with them.

In the beginning, most people feel odd because their natural food is off the table. When your menu consists of more fats and proteins, it is natural to feel that something is missing.

Your brain alarms you that you haven't eaten enough and sends you signals that you are hungry. It is literally "panicking" and telling you that you are starving, which is not correct. You get to eat, and you get to eat plenty of good food, but not carbs.

This condition usually arises during the first day or two. Afterward, people get used to their new eating habits. Once the brain "realizes" that carbs are no longer an option, it will focus on "finding" another abundant energy source: in this case, fats.

Not only is your food rich in fats, but your body contains stored fats in large amounts. As you consume more fats and fewer carbs, your body "runs" on the fats, both consumed and stored. The best thing is that, as the fats are used for energy, they are burned. This is how you get a double gain from this diet.

Usually, it will take a few days of consuming low-carb meals before you start seeing visible weight loss results.

You will not even have to check your weight because the fat layers will be visibly reduced.

This diet requires you to lower your daily consumption of carbs to only 20 grams. For most people, this transition from a regular carb-rich diet can be quite a challenge. Most people are used to eating bread, pasta, rice, dairy products, sweets, soda, alcohol, and fruits, so quitting all these foods might be challenging.

However, this is all in your head. If you manage to win the "battle" with your mind and endure the diet for a few days, you will see that you no longer have cravings as time goes by. Plus, the weight loss and the fat burn will be a great motivation to continue with this diet.

The keto diet practically makes the body burn fats much faster than carbohydrates; the foods you consume with this diet are quite rich in fats.

Carbs will be there, too, but at far lower levels than before. Foods rich in carbohydrates are the body's primary fuel or the brain's food. (Our bodies turn carbs into glucose.) Because there are hardly any carbohydrates in this diet, the body will have to find a substitute source of energy to keep itself alive.

Many people who don't truly need to lose weight and are completely healthy still choose to follow the keto diet because it is a great way to keep their meals balanced. Also, it is the perfect way to cleanse the body of toxins, processed foods, sugars, and unnecessary carbs. The combination of these things is usually the main reason for heart failure, some cancers, diabetes, cholesterol, or obesity.

If you ask a nutritionist about this diet, they will recommend it without a doubt. So, if you feel like cleansing your body and starting a diet that will keep you healthy, well-fed, and slender, perhaps the keto diet should be your primary choice.

And what is the best thing about it (besides the fact that you will balance your weight & lower the risk of many diseases)?

There is no yo-yo effect. The keto diet can be followed forever and has no side effects. It does not restrict you from following it for a few weeks or a month. Once you get your body to keto foods, you will not think about going back to the old ways of eating your meals.

Why No Carbs?

I don't hate carbs. They're one of nature's ways of fueling our bodies and brains. However, we eat far too much of this stuff by the way we live lately.

Mostly, in the form of processed sugars, refined carbs, and other high carb foods.

They spell disaster for your body, and you start piling on weight in those places you hate the most. In your stomach, your hips, your legs, your butt, your arms, your neck. Everywhere that's wrong! It leaves you more vulnerable to health problems such as type 2 diabetes, metabolic syndrome, depression and anxiety, certain cancers and just many more.

CHAPTER 2: Tips to Tackle Keto Diet

Successfully and with Serenity

Nobody told you that life was going to be this way! But don't worry. There's still plenty of time to make amendments and take care of your health. Here are a couple of tips that will allow you to lead a healthier life in your fifties:

Start Building on Immunity

Every day, our bod y is exposed to free radicals and toxins from the environment. The added stress of work and family problems doesn't make itany easier for us. To combat this, you must start consuming healthy veggies that contain plenty of antioxidants and build a healthier immune system.

This helps ward off unwanted illnesses and diseases, allowing you to maintain good health.

Adding more healthy veggies to your keto diet will help you obtain various minerals, vitamins, and antioxidants.

Consider Quitting Smoking

It's never too late to try to quit smoking, even if you are in your fifties. Once you start quitting, you'll notice how you'll be able to breathe easier while acquiring a better sense of smell and taste. Over a period of time, eliminating the habit of smoking can greatly reduce the risks of high blood pressure, strokes, and heart attack. Please note how these diseases are much more common among people in the fifties and above than in younger people.

Not to mention, quitting smoking will help you stay more active and enjoy better health with your friends and family.

Stay Social

Aging can be a daunting process, and trying to get through it all on your own isn't particularly helpful. We recommend you to stay in touch with friends and family or become a part of a local community club or network. Some older people find it comforting to get an emotional support animal.

Being surrounded by people you love will give you a sense of belonging and will improve your mood. It'll also keep your mind and memory sharp as you engage in different conversations.

Health Screenings You Should Get After Your Fifties

Your fifties are considered the prime years of your life. Don't let the joy of these years be robbed away from you because of poor health. Getting simple tests done can go a long way in identifying any potential health problems that you may have. Here's a list of health screenings you should get done:

Check Your Blood Pressure

Your blood pressure is a reliable indicator of your heart health. In simple words, blood pressure is a measure of how fast blood travels through the artery walls. Very high or even very low blood pressure can be a sign of an underlying problem. Once you reach your 40s, you should have your blood pressure checked more often.

EKG

The EKG reveals your heart health and activity. Short for electrocardiogram, the EKG helps identify problems in the heart. The process works by highlighting any rhythm problems that may be in the heart, such as poor heart muscles, improper blood flow, or any other form of abnormality. Getting an EKG is also a predictive measure for understanding the chances of a heart attack. Since people starting their fifties are at greater risk of getting a heart attack, you should get yourself checked more often.

Mammogram

Mammograms help rule out the risks of breast cancer. Women who enter their fifties should ideally get a mammogram after every ten years. However, if you have a family history, it is advisable that you get one much earlier to rule out cancer possibilities.

Blood Sugar Levels

If you're somebody who used to grab a fast-food meal every once in a while before you switched to keto, then you should definitely check your blood sugar levels more carefully. Blood sugar levels indicate whether or not you have diabetes. And you know how the saying goes, "prevention is better than." It's best to clear these possibilities out of the way sooner than later.

Check for Osteoporosis

Unfortunately, as you grow older, you also become susceptible to a number of bone diseases. Osteoporosis is a bone-related condition in which bones begin to lose mass, becoming frail and weak. Owing to this, seniors become more prone to fractures. This can make even the smallest of falls detrimental to your health.

Annual Physical Exam

Your insurance must be providing coverage for your annual physical exam.

So, there's no reason why you should not take advantage of it. This checkup helps identify the state of your health. You'll probably be surprised by how doctors can tell from a single blood test.

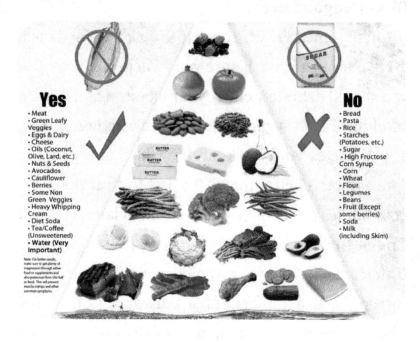

CHAPTER 3: Top Recipes

Pork Cutlets with Spanish Onion

Preparation time: 15 minutes

Cooking time: 15 minutes

Servings: 4

Ingredients:

- 1 tbsp. olive oil
- 2 pork cutlets
- 1 bell pepper, deveined and sliced
- 1 Spanish onion, chopped
- 2 garlic cloves, minced
- 1/2 tsp. hot sauce
- 1/2 tsp. mustard
- 1/2 tsp. paprika

Kitchen Equipment:

- Saucepan

Directions:

1. Fry the pork cutlets for 3 to 4 minutes until evenly golden and crispy on both sides.

2. Set the temperature to medium and add the bell pepper, Spanish onion, garlic, hot sauce, and mustard; continue cooking until the vegetables have softened, for a further 3 minutes.

3. Sprinkle with paprika, salt, and black pepper.

4. Serve immediately and enjoy!

Nutrition for Total Servings:

Calories: 403

Protein: 18.28 g

Fat: 24.1g

Carbs: 3.4g

Rich and Easy Pork Ragout

Preparation time: 15 minutes

Cooking time: 15 minutes

Servings: 4

Ingredients:

- 1 tsp. lard, melted at room temperature
- 3/4-pound pork butt, cut into bite-sized cubes
- 1 red bell pepper, deveined and chopped
- 1 poblano pepper, deveined and chopped
- 2 cloves garlic, pressed
- 1/2 cup leeks, chopped
- 1/2 tsp. mustard seeds
- 1/4 tsp. ground allspice
- 1/4 tsp. celery seeds
- 1 cup roasted vegetable broth
- 2 vine-ripe tomatoes, pureed

Kitchen Equipment:

- Stockpot

Directions:

1. Melt the lard in a stockpot over moderate heat. Once hot, cook the pork cubes for 4 to 6 minutes, occasionally stirring to ensure even cooking.

2. Then, stir in the vegetables and continue cooking until they are tender and fragrant. Add in the salt, pepper, mustard seeds, allspice, celery seeds, roasted vegetable broth, and tomatoes.

3. Reduce the heat to simmer. Let it simmer for 30 minutes longer or until everything is heated through. Ladle into individual bowls and serve hot. Bon appétit!

Nutrition for Total Servings:

Calories: 389

Protein: 23.17 g

Fat: 24.3g

Carbs: 5.4g

Pulled Pork with Mint

Preparation time: 20 minutes

Cooking time: 15 minutes

Servings: 2

Ingredients:

- 1 tsp. lard, melted at room temperature
- 3/4 pork Boston butt, sliced
- 2 garlic cloves, pressed
- 1/2 tsp. red pepper flakes, crushed
- 1/2 tsp. black peppercorns, freshly cracked
- Sea salt, to taste
- 2 bell peppers, deveined and sliced

Kitchen Equipment:

- Cast-iron skillet

Directions:

1. Melt the lard in a cast-iron skillet over a moderate flame. Once hot, brown the pork for 2 minutes per side until caramelized and crispy on the edges.

2. Set the temperature to medium-low and continue cooking for another 4 minutes, turning over periodically. Shred the pork with two forks and return to the skillet.

3. Add the garlic, red pepper, black peppercorns, salt, and bell pepper and continue cooking for a further 2 minutes or until the peppers are just tender and fragrant.

Nutrition for Total Servings:

6.42 g Carbs

370 Calories

21.9g Fat

34.9g Protein

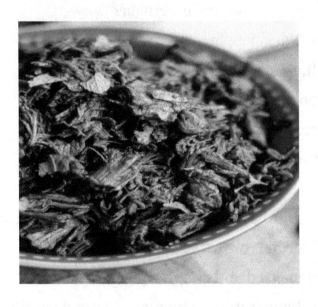

Festive Meatloaf

Preparation time: 1 hour

Cooking time: 50 minutes

Servings: 2

Ingredients:

- 1/4-pound ground pork
- 1/2-pound ground chuck
- 2 eggs, beaten
- 1/4 cup flaxseed meal
- 1 shallot, chopped
- 2 garlic cloves, minced
- 1/2 tsp. smoked paprika
- 1/4 tsp. dried basil
- 1/4 tsp. ground cumin
- Kosher salt, to taste
- 1/2 cup tomato puree
- 1 tsp. mustard
- 1 tsp. liquid monk fruit

Kitchen Equipment:

- 2 mixing bowl
- Loaf pan
- Oven

Directions:

1. In a bowl, mix the ground meat, eggs, flaxseed meal, shallot, garlic, and spices thoroughly.

2. In another bowl, mix the tomato puree with the mustard and liquid monk fruit, whisk to combine well.

3. Press the mixture into the loaf pan—Bake in the preheated oven at 360°F for 30 minutes.

Nutrition for Total Servings:

Carbs: 15.64 g

Calories: 517

Fat: 32.3g

Protein: 48.5g

Rich Winter Beef Stew

Preparation time: 45 minutes

Cooking time: 50 minutes

Servings: 2

Ingredients:

• 1-ounce bacon, diced

• 3/4-pound well-marbled beef chuck, boneless and cut into 1- 1/2-inch

pieces

• 1 red bell pepper, chopped

• 1 green bell pepper, chopped

• 2 garlic cloves, minced

• 1/2 cup leeks, chopped

• 1 parsnip, chopped

• Sea salt, to taste

• 1/4 tsp. mixed peppercorns, freshly cracked

• 2 cups of chicken bone broth

• 1 tomato, pureed

• 2 cups kale, torn into pieces

• 1 tbsp. fresh cilantro, roughly chopped

Kitchen Equipment:

• Dutch pot

Directions:

1. Heat a Dutch pot over medium-high flame. Now, cook the bacon until it is well browned and crisp; reserve. Then, cook the beef pieces for 3 to 5 minutes or until just browned on all sides; reserve. After that, sauté the peppers, garlic, leeks, and parsnip in the pan drippings until they are just tender and aromatic. Add the salt, peppercorns, chicken bone broth, tomato, and reserved beef to the pot. Bring to a boil. Stir in the kale leaves and continue simmering until the leaves have wilted or 3 to 4 minutes more.

2. Ladle into individual bowls & serve garnished with fresh cilantro and the reserved bacon.

Nutrition for Total Servings:

Carbs: 16.14 g

Protein: 88.75 g

Calories: 359

Fat: 17.8g

Mocha Crunch Oatmeal

Preparation time: 15 minutes

Cooking time: 5 minutes

Servings: 4

Ingredients:

• 1 cup of steel-cut oats

• 1 1/2 cup of cocoa powder

• 1/4 tsp. salt

• 2 cups of sugar

• 1/4 cup of agave nectar roasted mixed nuts

• 1/4 cup of bittersweet chocolate chips Milk or cream to serve.

• 2 tbsp. Fine espresso coffee

Kitchen Equipment:

• Saucepan

Directions:

1. Bring water to a boil. Stir in oats, cocoa powder, espresso, and salt.

Bring to a boil again and raising heat to medium-low.

Simmer uncovered for 20 to 30 minutes, frequently stirring until the oats hit the tenderness you need.

Remove from heat and whisk in sugar or agave nectar.

2. While the oatmeal cooks, the mixed nuts and chocolate chips roughly chop. Place them in a small bowl to eat.

3. Serve with hot oat milk or cream on the side when the oatmeal is full, and sprinkle liberally with a coating of nut and chocolate.

Nutrition for Total Servings:

Carbs: 111.9 g

Calories: 118

Fat: 12g

Protein: 26g

Keto Pancakes

Preparation time: 5 minutes

Cooking time: 15 minutes

Servings: 10

Ingredients:

- 1/2 c. almond flour
- Soy milk
- Four large eggs
- 1 tsp. lemon zest
- Butter, for frying and serving

Kitchen Equipment:

- Nonstick skillet

Directions:

1. Whisk almond flour, soy milk, eggs, and lemon zest together in a medium bowl until smooth.

2. Heat one tbsp. butter over medium flame in a non-stick skillet. Pour in the batter for about three tbsps., and cook for 2 minutes until golden. Flip over and cook for 2 minutes. Switch to a plate, and start with the batter remaining.

3. Serve with butter on top.

Nutrition for Total Servings:

Carbs: 0.14 g

Calories: 110

Fats: 10g

Protein: 28g

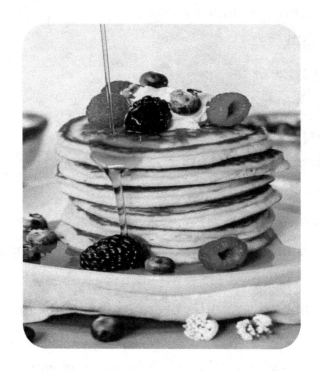

Keto Sausage Breakfast Sandwich

Preparation time: 5 minutes

Cooking time: 15 minutes

Servings: 3

Ingredients:

• 6 large eggs

• 2 tbsp. heavy cream

• Pinch red pepper flakes

• 1 tbsp. butter

• 6 frozen sausage patties, heated according to package instructions

• Avocado, sliced

Kitchen Equipment:

• Small bowl

• Nonstick container

Directions:

1. Beat the eggs, heavy cream, and red pepper flakes together in a small bowl.

4. Heat butter in a non-stick container over medium flame. Pour 1/3 of the eggs into your skillet. Allow it to sit for about 1 minute.

Fold the egg sides in the middle. Remove from saucepan and repeat with eggs left over.

2. Serve the eggs with avocado in between two sausage patties.

Nutrition for Total Servings:

Carbs: 42.17 g

Calories: 113

Fats: 10g

Protein: 27g

Crunchy Coconut Cluster Keto Cereal

Preparation time: 5 minutes

Cooking time: 20 minutes

Servings: 4

Ingredients:

• 1/2 cup of unsweetened shredded coconut

• 1/2 cup of hemp hearts

• 1/2 cup of raw pumpkin seeds

• A pinch of sea salt

• 2 scoops of perfect Keto MCT oil powder

• 1 white egg

• 1 tsp. of cinnamon

Directions:

1. The oven should be pre-heated to 350°F

2. A sheet pan should then be lined with parchment paper

3. Stir all dry ingredients in the bowl

4. Using a separate bowl, mix the white egg until it becomes frothy. Then, pour it slowly into the dry; mix

5. Transfer the mixture into a sheet of the pan and flatten to a thickness of 1/4 of an inch

6. Leave to bake for 15 minutes. After removal, use a spatula to break up the mass into chunks and allow to bake for more than 5 minutes.

7. Lastly, take it out of the oven and serve with your soy milk of choice. It can be stored for three days in an airtight container at room temperature

Nutrition for Total Servings:

Calories: 5258 Cal

Fat: 25 g

Carbs: 7 g

Protein: 9 g

Spinach

Preparation time: 5 minutes

Cooking time: 25 minutes

Servings: 8

Ingredients:

• 2 (10-ounce) packages of frozen spinach, thawed & drained

• 1 1/2 cups water, divided

• 1/4 cup sour cream

• Oat milk

• 2 tbsps. butter

• 1 tbsp. onion, minced

• 1 tbsp. garlic, minced

• 1 tbsp. fresh ginger, minced

• 2 tbsps. tomato puree

• 2 teaspoons curry powder

• 2 teaspoons garam masala powder

• 2 teaspoons ground coriander

• 2 teaspoons ground cumin

• 2 teaspoons ground turmeric

• 2 teaspoons red pepper flakes, crushed

• Salt, to taste

Directions:

1. Place spinach, 1/2 cup of water, and sour cream in a blender and pulse until pureed.

2. Transfer the spinach puree into a bowl and set aside.

3. In a large non-stick wok, melt butter over medium-low heat and sauté onion, garlic, ginger, tomato puree, spices, and salt for about 2–3 minutes.

4. Add the spinach puree and remaining water and stir to combine.

5. Adjust the heat to medium & cook for about 3–5 minutes.

6. Add oat milk and stir to combine.

7. Adjust heat to low & cook for about 10–15 minutes.

8. Serve hot.

Nutrition for Total Servings:

Calories: 121 Cal

Fat: 12 g

Carbs: 9 g

Protein: 4 g

CHAPTER 4: Breakfast and Smoothies

Classic Western Omelet

Preparation time: 5 minutes

Cooking time: 10 minutes

Servings: 1

Ingredients:

- 2 teaspoons coconut oil
- 3 large eggs, whisked
- 1 tbsp. heavy cream
- Salt and pepper
- 1/4 cup diced green pepper
- 1/4 cup diced yellow onion
- 1/4 cup diced ham

Directions:

1. In a small bowl, whisk the eggs, heavy cream, salt, and pepper.

2. Heat up 1 tsp. of coconut oil over medium heat in a small skillet.

3. Add the peppers and onions, then sauté the ham for 3 to 4 minutes.

4. Spoon the mixture in a cup, and heat the skillet with the remaining oil.

5. Pour in the whisked eggs & cook until the egg's bottom begins to set.

6. Tilt the pan and cook until almost set to spread the egg.

7. Spoon the ham and veggie mixture over half of the omelet and turn over.

8. Let cook the omelet until the eggs are set and then serve hot.

Nutrition for Total Servings:

Calories: 415

Fat: 32,5 g

Protein: 5 g

Carbs: 6,5 g

Sheet Pan Eggs with Ham and Pepper Jack

Preparation time: 5 minutes

Cooking time: 15 minutes

Servings: 6

Ingredients:

• 12 large eggs, whisked

• Salt and pepper

• 2 cups diced ham

• Oat milk

Directions:

1. Now, preheat the oven to 350°F and grease a rimmed baking sheet bwith cooking spray.

2. Whisk the eggs in a mixing bowl then add salt and pepper until frothy.

3. Stir in the ham and oat milk and mix until well combined.

4. Pour the mixture into baking sheets and spread it into an even layer.

5. Bake for 12 to 15 mins until the egg is set.

6. Let cool slightly then cut it into squares to serve.

Nutrition for Total Servings:

Calories: 235

Fat: 15g

Protein: 21g

Carbs: 2.5g

Nutty Pumpkin Smoothie

Preparation time: 5 minutes

Cooking time: None

Servings: 1

Ingredients:

- 1 cup unsweetened soy milk
- 1/2 cup pumpkin puree
- 1/4 cup heavy cream
- 1 tbsp. raw almonds
- 1/4 tsp. pumpkin pie spice
- Liquid stevia extract, to taste

Directions:

1. Combine the ingredients in a blender.

2. Pulse the ingredients several times, then blend until smooth.

3. Pour into a large glass & enjoy immediately.

Nutrition for Total Servings:

Calories: 205

Fat: 16.5g

Protein: 3g

Carbs: 13g

Tomato Mozzarella Egg Muffins

Preparation time: 5 minutes

Cooking time: 25 minutes

Servings: 12

Ingredients:

- 1 tbsp. butter
- 1 medium tomato, finely diced
- 1/2 cup diced yellow onion
- 12 large eggs, whisked
- 1/2 cup of canned oat milk
- 1/4 cup sliced green onion
- Salt and pepper
- Soy milk

Directions:

1. Now, preheat the oven to 350°F and grease the cooking spray into a muffin pan.

2. Melt the butter over moderate heat in a medium skillet.

3. Add the tomato and onions, then cook until softened for 3 to 4 minutes.

4. Divide the mix between cups of muffins.

5. Whisk the bacon, oat milk, green onions, salt, and pepper together and then spoon into the muffin cups.

6. Sprinkle with soy milk until the egg is set, then bake for 15 to 25 minutes.

Nutrition for Total Servings:

Calories: 135

Fat: 10.5 g

Protein: 9 g

Carbs: 2 g

Crispy Chai Waffles

Preparation time: 10 minutes

Cooking time: 20 minutes

Servings: 4

Ingredients:

- 4 large eggs, and then separated in whites and yolks
- 3 tbsps. coconut flour
- 3 tbsps. powdered erythritol
- 1 1/4 tsp. baking powder
- 1 tsp. cocoa
- 1/2 tsp. ground cinnamon
- Pinch ground cloves
- Pinch ground cardamom
- 3 tbsps. coconut oil, melted
- 3 tbsps. unsweetened soy milk

Directions:

1. Divide the eggs into two separate mixing bowls.

2. Whip the whites of the eggs until stiff peaks develop and then set aside.

3. Whisk the egg yolks into the other bowl with the coconut flour,

erythritol, baking powder, cocoa, cinnamon, cardamom, and cloves.

4. Pour the melted coconut oil and the soy milk into the second bowl and whisk.

5. Fold softly in the whites of the egg until you have just combined.

6. Preheat waffle iron with cooking spray and grease.

7. Spoon into the iron for about 1/2 cup of batter.

8. Cook the waffle according to directions from the maker.

9. Move the waffle to a plate and repeat with the batter leftover.

Nutrition for Total Servings:

Calories: 215

Fat: 17 g

Protein: 8 g

Carbs: 8 g

Broccoli, Kale, Egg Scramble

Preparation time: 5 minutes

Cooking time: 10 minutes

Servings: 1

Ingredients:

- 2 large eggs, whisked
- 1 tbsp. heavy cream
- Salt and pepper
- 1 tsp. coconut oil
- 1 cup fresh chopped kale
- 1/4 cup frozen broccoli florets, thawed
- Soy milk
- 1/3 cup parmesan cheese

Directions:

1. In a mug, whisk the eggs along with the heavy cream, salt, and pepper.

2. Heat 1 tsp. coconut oil over medium heat in a medium-size skillet.

3. Stir in the kale & broccoli, then cook about 1 to 2 minutes until the kale is wilted.

4. Pour in the eggs and cook until just set, stirring occasionally.

5. Stir in the soy milk with parmesan and serve hot.

Nutrition for Total Servings:

Calories: 315

Fat: 23 g

Protein: 19.5 g

Carbs: 10 g

CHAPTER 5: Appetizers and Snacks Recipes

Baked Chorizo

Preparation time: 10 minutes

Cooking time: 30 minutes

Servings: 6

Ingredients:

7 oz. Spanish chorizo, sliced

1/4 cup chopped parsley

Directions:

1. Now, preheat the oven to 325 F. Line a baking dish with waxed paper. Bake the chorizo for minutes until crispy. Remove from the oven and let cool.

2. Arrange on a servings platter. Top each slice and parsley.

Nutrition for Total Servings:

Calories: 172

Carbs: 0.2g

Fat: 13g

Protein: 5g

Caribbean-Style Chicken Wings

Preparation time: 10 minutes

Cooking time: 50 minutes

Servings: 2

Ingredients:

- 4 chicken wings
- 1 tbsp. coconut aminos
- 2 tbsps. rum
- 2 tbsps. butter
- 1 tbsp. onion powder
- 1 tbsp. garlic powder
- 1/2 tsp. salt
- 1/4 tsp. freshly ground black pepper
- 1/2 tsp. red pepper flakes
- 1/4 tsp. dried dill
- 2 tbsps. sesame seeds

Directions:

1. Pat dry the chicken wings. Toss the chicken wings with the remaining ingredients until well coated. Arrange the chicken wings on a parchment-lined baking sheet.

2. Bake in the preheated oven at 200°F for 45 minutes until golden brown.

3. Serve with your favorite sauce for dipping. Bon appétit!

Nutrition for Total Servings:

Calories: 18.5g

Fat: 5.2g

Carbs: 15.6g

Protein: 1.9g

Rosemary Chips with Guacamole

Preparation time: 10 minutes

Cooking time: 20 minutes

Servings: 4

Ingredients:

- 1 tbsp. rosemary
- 1/4 tsp. garlic powder
- 2 avocados, pitted and scooped
- 1 tomato, chopped
- 1 tsp. salt

Directions:

1. Now, preheat the oven to 350 F and line a baking sheet with parchment paper. Mix, rosemary, and garlic powder evenly.

2. Spoon 6-8 teaspoons on the baking sheet creating spaces between each mound.

3. Flatten mounds. Bake for 5 minutes, cool, and remove to a plate. To in tomato and continue to mash until mostly smooth. Season with salt.

4. Serve crackers with guacamole.

Nutrition for Total Servings:

Calories: 229

Net Carbs: 2g

Fat: 20g

Protein: 10g

Golden Crisps

Preparation time: 10 minutes

Cooking time: 10 minutes

Servings: 4

Ingredients:

• 1/3 tsp. dried oregano

• 1/3 tsp. dried rosemary

• 1/2 tsp. garlic powder

• 1/3 tsp. dried basil

Directions:

1. Now, preheat the oven to 390°F.

2. In a small bowl mix the dried oregano, rosemary, basil, and garlic powder. Set aside.

3. Line a large baking dish with parchment paper. Sprinkle with the dry seasonings mixture and bake for 6-7 minutes.

4. Let cool for a few minutes and enjoy.

Nutrition for Total Servings:

Calories: 296

Fat: 22.7g

Carbs: 1.8g

Protein: 22g

Butternut Squash & Spinach Stew

Preparation time: 10 minutes

Cooking time: 35 minutes

Servings: 4

Ingredients:

• 2 tbsps. olive oil

• 1 Spanish onion, peeled and diced

• 1 garlic clove, minced

• 1/2 pound butternut squash, diced

• 1 celery stalk, chopped

• 3 cups vegetable broth

• Kosher salt and freshly cracked black pepper, to taste

• 4 cups baby spinach

• 4 tbsps. sour cream

Directions:

1. Now, preheat the oven olive oil in a soup pot over a moderate flame. Now, sauté the Spanish onion until tender and translucent.

2. Then, cook the garlic until just tender and aromatic.

3. Stir in the butternut squash, celery, broth, salt, and black pepper. Turn the heat to simmer and let it cook, covered, for minutes.

4. Fold in the baby spinach leaves and cover with the lid; let it sit in the residual heat until the baby spinach wilts completely.

5. Serve dolloped with cold sour cream. Enjoy!

Nutrition for Total Servings:

Calories: 148

Fat: 11.5g

Carbs: 6.8g

Protein: 2.5g

Italian-Style Asparagus

Preparation time: 10 minutes

Cooking time: 10 minutes

Servings: 2

Ingredients:

• 1/2 pound asparagus spears, trimmed, cut into bite-sized pieces

• 1 tsp. Italian spice blend

• 1/2 tbsp. lemon juice

• 1 tbsp. extra-virgin olive oil

Directions:

1. Bring a saucepan of lightly salted water to a boil. Turn the heat to medium-low. Add the asparagus spears and cook for approximately 3 minutes. Drain and transfer to a serving bowl.

2. Add the Italian spice blend, lemon juice, and extra-virgin olio e oil; toss until well coated.

3. Serve immediately. Bon appétit!

Nutrition for Total Servings:

Calories: 193

Fat: 14.1g

Carbs: 5.6g

Protein: 11.5g

Crunchy Rutabaga Puffs

Preparation time: 10 minutes

Cooking time: 35 minutes

Servings: 4

Ingredients:

- 1 rutabaga, peeled and diced
- 2 tbsp. melted butter
- 1/4 cup ground pork rinds
- Pinch of salt and black pepper

Directions:

1. Now, preheat the oven to 400 F and spread rutabaga on a baking sheet. Season with salt, pepper, and drizzle with butter.

2. Bake until tender, minutes. Transfer to a bowl. Allow cooling. Using a fork, mash and mix the ingredients.

3. Pour the pork rinds onto a plate. Mold 1-inch balls out of the rutabaga mixture and roll properly in the rinds while pressing gently to stick. Place on the same baking sheet and bake for 10 minutes until golden.

Nutrition for Total Servings:

Calories: 129

Carbs: 5.9g

Fat: 8g

Protein: 3g

Spinach & Chicken Meatballs

Preparation time: 10 minutes

Cooking time: 30 minutes

Servings: 10

Ingredients:

- 1 tbsp. Italian seasoning mix
- 1 1/2 pounds ground chicken
- 1 tsp. garlic, minced
- 1 egg, whisked
- 8 ounces spinach, chopped
- 1/2 tsp. mustard seeds
- Sea salt and ground black pepper, to taste
- 1/2 tsp. paprika

Directions:

1. Mix the ingredients until everything is well incorporated.

2. Now, shape the meat mixture into meatballs. Transfer your meatballs to a baking sheet and brush them with nonstick cooking oil.

3. Bake in the preheated oven at 200°F for about 25 minutes or until golden brown. Serve with cocktail sticks and enjoy!

Nutrition for Total Servings:

Calories: 207

Fat: 12.3g

Carbs: 4.4

Protein: 19.5g

Herbed Coconut Flour Bread

Preparation time: 10 minutes

Cooking time: 3 minutes

Servings: 2

Ingredients:

- 4 tbsp. coconut flour
- 1/2 tsp. baking powder
- 1/2 tsp. dried thyme
- 2 tbsp. whipping cream
- 2 eggs

Seasoning:

- 1/2 tsp. oregano
- 2 tbsp. avocado oil

Directions:

1. Take a medium bowl, place all the ingredients in it and then whisk until incorporated and smooth batter comes together.

2. Distribute the mixture evenly between two mugs and then microwave for a minute and 30 seconds until cooked.

3. When done, take out bread from the mugs, cut it into slices, and then serve.

Nutrition for Total Servings:

Calories: 309

Fats: 26.1 g

Protein: 9.3 g

Carb: 4.3 g

Minty Zucchinis

Preparation time: 10 minutes

Cooking time: 15 minutes

Servings: 4

Ingredients:

- 1 pound zucchinis, sliced
- 1 tbsp. olive oil
- 2 garlic cloves, minced
- 1 tbsp. mint, chopped
- Pinch of salt and black pepper
- 1/4 cup veggie stock

Directions:

1. Heat up a pan with the oil over medium-high heat, add the garlic and sauté for 2 minutes.

2. Add the zucchinis and the other ingredients, toss, cook everything for 10 minutes more, divide between plates and serve as a side dish.

Nutrition for Total Servings:

Calories: 70

Fat: 1g

Carbs: 0.4g

Protein: 6g

CHAPTER 6: Soup and Stew Recipes

Hearty Fall Stew

Preparation time: 15 minutes

Cooking time: 8 hrs.

Servings: 6

Ingredients:

- 3 tbsps. extra-virgin olive oil, divided
- 1 (2-pound/907-g) beef chuck roast, cut into 1-inch chunks
- 1/2 tsp. salt
- 1/4 tsp. freshly ground black pepper
- 1/4 cup apple cider vinegar
- 1/2 sweet onion, chopped
- 1 cup diced tomatoes
- 1 tsp. dried thyme
- 1 1/2 cups pumpkin, cut into 1-inch chunks
- 2 cups beef broth
- 2 teaspoons minced garlic
- 1 tbsp. chopped fresh parsley, for garnish

Directions:

1. Add beef to the skillet, and sprinkle salt and pepper to season.

2. Cook the beef for 7 minutes or until well browned.

3. Put the cooked beef into the slow cooker and add the remaining ingredients, except for the parsley, to the slow cooker. Stir to mix well.

4. Slow cook for 8 hrs. And top with parsley before serving.

Nutrition for Total Servings:

Calories: 462

Fat: 19.1g

Carbs: 10.7 g

Protein: 18.6 g

Chicken Mushroom Soup

Preparation time: 15 minutes

Cooking time: 10-15 minutes

Servings: 4

Ingredients:

- 6 cups of chicken stock
- 5 slices of chopped bacon
- 4 cups cooked chicken breast, chopped
- 3 cups of water
- 2 cups of chopped celery root
- 2 cups of sliced yellow squash
- 2 tbsps. of olive oil
- 1/2 tsp. of avocado oil
- 1/4 cup of chopped basil
- 1/4 cup of chopped onion
- 1/4 cup of chopped tomatoes
- 1 tbsp. of ground garlic
- 1 cup of sliced white mushrooms
- 1 cup green beans
- Salt
- Black pepper

Directions:

1. Heat oil in a skillet, add in half of the onions, sauté until soft.

2. Put in bacon and fry for a minute and a half.

3. Then, add in onions, garlic, tomatoes, and mushrooms, stir fry for three minutes.

4. Put in stock and fat water with the rest of the ingredients. Let it simmer for 10-15 minutes. Serve hot.

Nutrition for Total Servings:

Calories: 268

Fat: 10.5g

Carbs: 3.1 g

Protein: 12.9g

Cold Green Beans and Avocado Soup

Preparation time: 15 minutes

Cooking time: 15 minutes

Servings: 4

Ingredients:

- 1 tbsp. butter
- 2 tbsp. almond oil
- 1 garlic clove, minced
- 1 cup (227 g) green beans (fresh or frozen)
- 1/4 avocado
- 1 cup heavy cream
- 1/2 tsp. coconut aminos
- Salt to taste

Directions:

1. Now, preheat the oven butter and almond oil in a large skillet and sauté the garlic for 30 seconds.

2. Add the green beans and stir-fry for 10 minutes or until tender.

3. Add the mixture to a food processor and top with the avocado, heavy cream, coconut aminos, and salt.

4. Blend the ingredients until smooth.

5. Pour the soup into serving bowls, cover with plastic wraps and chill in the fridge for at least 2 hours.

Nutrition for Total Servings:

Calories: 301

Fat: 3.1g

Carbs: 2.8 g

Protein: 3.1g

Creamy Mixed Seafood Soup

Preparation time: 15 minutes

Cooking time: 15 minutes

Servings: 4

Ingredients:

- 1 tbsp. avocado oil
- 2 garlic cloves, minced
- 3/4 tbsp. almond flour
- 1 cup vegetable broth
- 1 tsp. dried dill
- 1 lb. frozen mixed seafood
- Salt and black pepper to taste
- 1 tbsp. plain vinegar
- 2 cups cooking cream
- Fresh dill leaves to garnish

Directions:

1. Heat oil sauté the garlic for 30 seconds or until fragrant.

2. Stir in the almond flour until brown.

3. Mix in the vegetable broth until smooth and stir in the dill, seafood mix, salt, and black pepper.

4. Bring soup to a boil and then simmer for 3 to 4 minutes or until the seafood cooks.

5. Add the vinegar, cooking cream, and stir well. Garnish with dill, serve.

Nutrition for Total Servings:

Calories: 361

Fat: 12.4g

Carbs: 3.9 g

Protein: 11.7g

Roasted Tomato and Cheddar Soup

Preparation time: 10 minutes

Cooking time: 15-20 minutes

Servings: 4

Ingredients:

- 2 tbsp. butter
- 2 medium yellow onions, sliced
- 4 garlic cloves, minced
- 5 thyme sprigs
- 8 basil leaves + extra for garnish
- 8 tomatoes
- 1/2 tsp. red chili flakes
- 2 cups vegetable broth
- Salt and black pepper to taste

Directions:

1. Melt the butter in a pot and sauté the onions and garlic for 3 minutes or until softened.

2. Stir in the thyme, basil, tomatoes, red chili flakes, and vegetable broth.

3. Season with salt and black pepper.

4. Boil it then simmer for 10 minutes or until the tomatoes soften.

5. Puree all ingredients until smooth. Season.

6. Garnish with the basil. Serve warm.

Nutrition for Total Servings:

Calories: 341

Fat: 12.9g

Carbs: 4.8 g

Protein: 4.1g

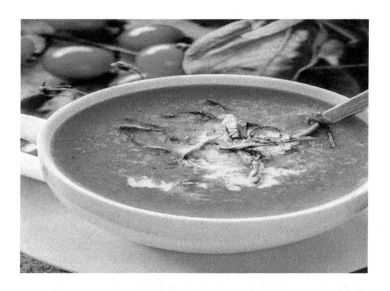

Cauliflower Kale Soup

Preparation time: 10 minutes

Cooking time: 50 minutes

Servings: 4

Ingredients:

• 4 cups cauliflower florets

• 6 cups vegetable stock

• 1 tbsp. garlic, minced

• 1/4 cup onion, chopped

• 6 oz. kale, chopped

• 6 tbsp. olive oil

• Pepper

• Salt

Directions:

1. Now, preheat the oven to 425 F.

2. Spread cauliflower onto the baking tray and drizzle with two tbsps. Of oil and season with pepper and salt.

3. Roast cauliflower in a preheated oven for 25 minutes. Remove from the oven and set aside.

4. In a bowl, toss kale with two tbsps. Of oil and season with salt. Arrange kale onto the baking tray and bake at 300 F for 30 minutes. Toss halfway through.

5. Heat oil.

6. Add onion and sauté for 3-4 minutes. Add garlic and sauté for a minute.

7. Add stock and roasted cauliflower and bring to boil.

8. Simmer it for 10 minutes.

9. Add kale and cook for 10 minutes more.

10. Puree the soup until smooth.

11. Serve and enjoy.

Nutrition for Total Servings:

Calories: 287

Fat: 15.1g

Carbs: 3.1 g

Protein: 5.8g

Healthy Celery Soup

Preparation time: 10 minutes

Cooking time: 20 minutes

Servings: 4

Ingredients:

• 3 cups celery, chopped

• 1 cup vegetable broth

• 1 1/2 tbsp. fresh basil, chopped

• 1/4 cup onion, chopped

• 1 tbsp. garlic, chopped

• 1 tbsp. olive oil

• 1/4 tsp. pepper

• 1/2 tsp. salt

Directions:

1. Heat some oil.

2. Add celery, onion & garlic to the saucepan and sauté for 4-5 minutes or until softened.

3. Add broth and bring to boil. Turn heat to low and simmer.

4. Add basil.

5. Season soup with pepper and salt.

6. Puree the soup until smooth.

7. Serve and enjoy.

Nutrition for Total Servings:

Calories: 201

Fat: 5.4g

Carbs: 3.9 g

Protein: 5.1g

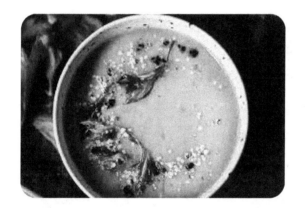

Creamy Asparagus Soup

Preparation time: 10 minutes

Cooking time: 15 minutes

Servings: 4

Ingredients:

• 2 lbs. asparagus, cut the ends and chop into 1/2-inch pieces

• 2 tbsp. olive oil

• 3 garlic cloves, minced

• 1/2 cup heavy cream

• 1/4 cup onion, chopped

• 4 cups vegetable stock

• Pepper

• Salt

Directions:

1. Heat olive oil in large pot over medium heat.

2. Add onion to the pot and sauté until onion is softened.

3. Add asparagus and sauté for 2-3 minutes.

4. Add garlic and sauté for a minute. Season with pepper and salt.

5. Add stock and bring to boil. Turn heat to low and simmer until asparagus is tender.

6. Remove pot from heat and puree the soup using an immersion blender until creamy.

7. Return pot on heat. Add cream and stir well and cook over medium heat until just soup is hot. Do not boil the soup.

8. Remove from heat.

9. Serve and enjoy.

Nutrition for Total Servings:

Calories: 202

Fat: 8.4g

Carbs: 3.1g

Protein: 5.3g

CHAPTER 7: Desserts Recipes

Mocha Mousse

Preparation time: 2 hours and 35 minutes

Cooking time: 0 minutes

Servings: 4

Ingredients:

- 3 tbsps. sour cream, full-fat
- 2 tbsps. butter, softened
- 1 1/2 teaspoons vanilla extract, unsweetened
- 1/3 cup erythritol
- 1/4 cup cocoa powder, unsweetened
- 3 teaspoons instant coffee powder

For the Whipped Cream:

- 2/3 cup heavy whipping cream, full-fat
- 1 1/2 tsp. erythritol
- 1/2 tsp. vanilla extract, unsweetened

Directions:

1. Add sour cream and butter then beat until smooth.

2. Now add erythritol, cocoa powder, coffee, and vanilla and blend until incorporated, set aside until required.

3. Prepare whipping cream: For this, place whipping cream in a bowl and beat until soft peaks form.

4. Beat in vanilla and erythritol until stiff peaks form, and fold until just mixed.

5. Then add remaining whipping cream mixture and fold until evenly incorporated.

6. Spoon the mousse into a freezer-proof bowl and place in the refrigerator for 2 1/2 hours until set.

7. Serve straight away.

Nutrition for Total Servings:

Calories: 421.7

Fat: 42 g

Protein: 6 g

Carbs: 6.5 g

Pumpkin Pie Pudding

Preparation time: 4 hours and 25 minutes

Cooking time: 20 minutes

Servings: 4

Ingredients:

- 2 eggs
- 1 cup heavy whipping cream, divided
- 3/4 cup erythritol sweetener
- 15 ounces pumpkin puree
- 1 tsp. pumpkin pie spice
- 1 tsp. vanilla extract, unsweetened
- 1 1/2 cup water

Directions:

1. Crack eggs in a bowl, add 1/2 cup cream, sweetener, pumpkin puree, pumpkin pie spice, and vanilla and whisk until blended.

2. Take a 6 by 3-inch baking pan, grease it well with avocado oil, then pour in egg mixture, smooth the top and cover with aluminum foil.

3. Switch on the instant pot, pour in water, insert a trivet stand and place baking pan on it.

4. Shut the instant pot with its lid in the sealed position, then press the 'manual' button, press '+/-' to the set the

cooking time to 20 minutes & cook at high-pressure setting; when the pressure builds in the pot, the cooking timer will start.

5. When the instant pot buzzes, press the 'keep warm' button, release pressure naturally for 10 min, and then do quick pressure release and open the lid.

6. Take out the baking pan, uncover it, let cool for 15 minutes at room temperature, then transfer the pan into the refrigerator for 4 hours or until cooled.

7. Top pie with remaining cream, then cut it into slices and serve.

Nutrition for Total Servings:

Calories: 184

Fat: 16 g

Protein: 3 g

Carbs: 5 g

Avocado & Chocolate Pudding

Preparation time: 20 minutes

Cooking time: 10 minutes

Servings: 2

Ingredients:

- 1 ripe medium avocado
- 1 tsp. natural sweetener
- 1/4 tsp. vanilla extract
- 4 tbsp. unsweetened cocoa powder
- 1 pinch pink salt

Directions:

1. Combine the avocado, sweetener, vanilla, cocoa powder, and salt into the blender or processor.

2. Pulse until creamy smooth.

3. Measure into fancy dessert dishes and chill for at least 1/2 hour.

Nutrition for Total Servings:

Calories: 281

Carbs: 2 g

Protein: 8 g

Fat: 27 g

Cake Pudding

Preparation time: 5 min

Cooking time: 5 min

Servings: 4

Ingredients:

- ½ heavy whipping cream
- 1 tsp. lemon juice
- ½ sour cream
- 20 drops liquid stevia
- 1 tsp. vanilla extract

Directions:

1. Whip the sour cream and whipping cream together with the mixer until soft peaks form. Combine with the rest of the ingredients and whip until fluffy.

2. Portion into four dishes to chill. Place a layer of the wrap over the dish and store in the fridge.

3. When ready to eat, garnish with some berries if you like.

4. Note: If you add berries, be sure to add the carbs.

Nutrition for Total Servings:

Calories: 356

Carbs: 5 g

Protein: 5 g

Fat: 36 g

Carrot Almond Cake

Preparation time: 45 minutes

Cooking time: 15 minutes

Servings: 8

Ingredients:

• 3 eggs

• 1 ½ tsp. apple pie spice

• 1 cup almond flour

• 2/3 cup swerve

• 1 tsp. baking powder

• 1/4 cup coconut oil

• 1 cup shredded carrots

• 1/2 cup heavy whipping cream

• 1/2 cup chopped walnuts

Directions:

1. Grease cake pan. Combine all of the ingredients with the mixer until well mixed. Pour the mix into the pan and cover with a layer of foil.

2. Pour two cups of water into the Instant Pot bowl along with the steamer rack. Arrange the pan on the trivet and set the pot using the cake buttoo min.).

4. Natural-release the pressure for ten minutes. Then, quick-release the rest of the built-up steam pressure.

5. Cool then start frosting or serve it plain.

Nutrition for Total Servings:

Calories: 268

Carbs: 4 g

Fat: 25 g

Protein: 6 g

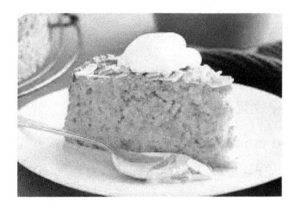

Chocolate Lava Cake

Preparation time: 20 minutes

Cooking time: 10 minutes

Servings: 4

Ingredients:

- ½ cup unsweetened cocoa powder
- ¼ cup melted butter
- 4 eggs
- ¼ tsp. sugar-free chocolate sauce
- ½ tsp. sea salt
- ½ tsp. ground cinnamon
- Pure vanilla extract
- ¼ cup Stevia
- Also Needed: Ice cube tray & 4 ramekins

Directions:

1. Pour one tbsp. of the chocolate sauce into four of the tray slots and freeze.

2. Warm up the oven to 350°Fahrenheit. Lightly grease the ramekins with butter or a spritz of oil.

3. Mix salt, cinnamon, cocoa powder, & stevia until combined. Whisk in the eggs – one at a time. Stir in the melted vanilla extract
and butter.

4. Fill each of the ramekins halfway & add one of the frozen chocolates. Cover the rest of the container with the cake batter.

5. Bake 13-14 min. When they're set, place on a wire rack to cool for about five minutes. Remove and put on a serving dish.

6. Enjoy by slicing its molten center.

Nutrition for Total Servings:

Calories: 189

Carbs: 3 g

Protein: 8 g

Fat: 17 g

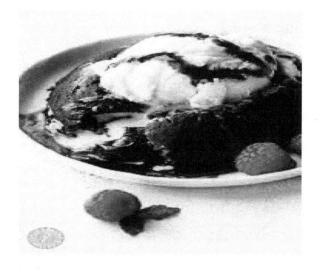

Glazed Pound Cake

Preparation time: 1 hour

Cooking time: 1 hours

Servings: 16

Ingredients:

- ½ tsp. salt
- 2 ½ cup almond flour
- ½ cup unsalted butter
- 1 ½ cup erythritol
- 8 unchilled eggs
- ½ tsp. lemon extract
- 1 ½ tsp. vanilla extract
- 1 ½ tsp. baking powder

The Glaze:

- ¼ cup powdered erythritol
- 3 tbsp. heavy whipping cream
- ½ tsp. vanilla extract

Directions:

1. Warm the oven to 350°Fahrenheit.

2. Whisk together baking powder, almond flour, and salt

3. Cream the erythritol, butter. Mix until smooth in a large mixing container.

4. Whisk and add the eggs with the lemon and vanilla extract. Blend with the rest of the ingredients using a hand mixer until smooth.

5. Dump the batter into a loaf pan. Bake for one to two hours.

6. Prepare a glaze. Mix in vanilla extract, powdered erythritol, and heavy whipping cream until smooth.

7. You should let the cake cool completely before adding the glaze.

Nutrition for Total Servings:

Calories: 254

Carbs: 2.5 g

Protein: 7.9 g

Fat: 23.4 g

CHAPTER 16: Drinks Recipes

Bulletproof Coffee

Preparation time: 5 minutes

Cooking time: 0 minutes

Servings: 1

Ingredients:

• 1 1/2 cups hot coffee

• 2 tbsps. MCT oil powder or Bulletproof Brain Octane Oil

• 2 tbsps. butter or ghee

Directions:

1. Pour the hot coffee into the blender.

2. Add the oil powder and butter, and blend until thoroughly mixed and frothy.

3. Pour into a large mug and enjoy.

Nutrition for Total Servings:

Calories: 245

Fat: 9.4g

Carbs: 1.2 g

Protein: 2.3g

Morning Berry-Green Smoothie

Preparation time: 15 minutes

Cooking time: 0 minutes

Servings: 4

Ingredients:

- 1 avocado, pitted and sliced
- 3 cups mixed blueberries and strawberries
- 2 cups unsweetened oat milk
- 6 tbsp. heavy cream
- 2 tsp. erythritol
- 1 cup of ice cubes
- 1/3 cup nuts and seeds mix

Directions:

1. Combine the avocado slices, blueberries, strawberries, oat milk, heavy cream, erythritol, ice cubes, nuts, and seeds in a smoothie maker; blend in high-speed until smooth and uniform.

2. Pour the smoothie into drinking glasses, and serve immediately.

Nutrition for Total Servings:

Calories: 290

Fat: 5.1g

Carbs: 1.4 g

Protein: 2g

Dark Chocolate Smoothie

Preparation time: 10 minutes

Cooking time: 0 minutes

Servings: 2

Ingredients:

- 8 pecans
- 3/4 cup of oat milk
- 1/4 cup of water
- 1 1/2 cups watercress
- 2 tsp. vegan protein powder
- 1 tbsp. chia seeds
- 1 tbsp. unsweetened cocoa powder
- 4 fresh dates, pitted

Directions:

1. In a blender, all ingredients must be blended until creamy and uniform.

2. Place into two glasses and chill before serving.

Nutrition for Total Servings:

Calories: 299

Fat: 10g

Carbs: 2.1 g

Protein: 4.4g

Super Greens Smoothie

Preparation time: 15 minutes

Cooking time: 0 minutes

Servings: 2

Ingredients:

• 6 kale leaves, chopped

• 3 stalks celery, chopped

• 1 ripe avocado, skinned, pitted, sliced

• 1 cup of ice cubes

• 2 cups spinach, chopped

• 1 large cucumber, peeled and chopped

• Chia seeds to garnish

Directions:

1. In a blender, add the kale, celery, avocado, and ice cubes, and blend for 45 seconds. Add the spinach and cucumber, and process for another 45 seconds until smooth.

2. Pour the smoothie into glasses, garnish it with chia seeds, and serve the drink immediately.

Nutrition for Total Servings:

Calories: 290

Fat: 9.4g

Carbs: 3.1 g

Protein: 8.5g

Kiwi Coconut Smoothie

Preparation time: 5 minutes
Cooking time: 0 minutes
Servings: 2
Ingredients:

- 2 kiwis, pulp scooped
- 1 tbsp. xylitol
- 4 ice cubes
- 2 cups unsweetened soy milk
- 1 cup of coconut yogurt
- Mint leaves to garnish

Directions:

1. Process the kiwis, xylitol, soy milk, yogurt, and ice cubes in a blender, until smooth, for about 3 minutes.
2. Transfer to serving glasses, garnish with mint leaves and serve.

Nutrition for Total Servings:

Calories: 298

Fat: 1.2g

Carbs: 1.2 g

Protein: 3.2g

Avocado-Coconut Shake

Preparation time: 5 minutes

Cooking time: 0 minutes

Servings: 2

Ingredients:

• 3 cups soy milk, chilled

• 1 avocado, pitted, peeled, sliced

• 2 tbsp. erythritol

• Coconut cream for topping

Directions:

1. Combine soy milk, avocado, and erythritol, into the smoothie maker, and blend for 1 minute to smooth.

2. Pour the drink into serving glasses, add some coconut cream on top of them, and garnish with mint leaves. Serve immediately.

Nutrition for Total Servings:

Calories: 301

Fat: 6.4g

Carbs: 0.4 g

Protein: 3.1g

Creamy Vanilla Cappuccino

Preparation time: 5 minutes

Cooking time: 0 minutes

Servings: 2

Ingredients:

• 2 cups unsweetened vanilla soy milk, chilled

• 1 tsp. swerve sugar

• 1/2 tbsp. powdered coffee

• 1/2 tsp. vanilla bean paste

• 1/4 tsp. xanthan gum

• Unsweetened chocolate shavings to garnish

Directions:

1. In a blender, combine the soy milk, swerve sugar, coffee, vanilla bean paste, and xanthan gum and process on high speed for 1 minute until smooth.

2. Pour into tall shake glasses, sprinkle with chocolate shavings, and serve immediately.

Nutrition for Total Servings:

Calories: 190

Fat: 4.1g

Carbs: 0.5 g

Protein: 2g

Golden Turmeric Latte with Nutmeg

Preparation time: 5 minutes

Cooking time: 5 minutes

Servings: 2

Ingredients:

• 2 cups oat milk

• 1/3 tsp. cinnamon powder

• 1/2 cup brewed coffee

• 1/4 tsp. turmeric powder

• 1 tsp. xylitol

• Nutmeg powder to garnish

Directions:

1. Add the oat milk, cinnamon powder, coffee, turmeric and xylitol to the blender.

2. Blend the ingredients at medium speed for 50 seconds and pour the mixture into a saucepan.

3. Over low heat, set the pan and heat through for 6 minutes, without boiling.

4. Keep swirling the pan to prevent boiling. Turn the heat off, and serve in latte cups, topped with nutmeg powder.

Nutrition for Total Servings:

Calories: 254

Fat: 9.1g

Carbs: 1.2g

Protein: 1 g

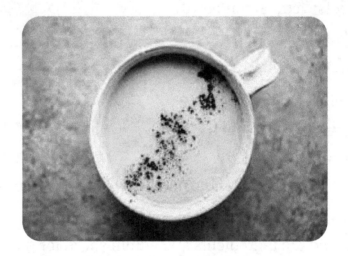

Almond Smoothie

Preparation time: 5 minutes

Cooking time: 0 minutes

Servings: 2

Ingredients:

- 2 cups soy milk
- 2 tbsp. almond butter
- 1/2 cup Greek yogurt
- 1 tsp. almond extract
- 1 tsp. cinnamon
- 4 tbsp. flax meal
- 30 drops of stevia
- A handful of ice cubes

Directions:

1. Put the yogurt, soy milk, almond butter, flax meal, almond extract, and stevia in the bowl of a blender.

2. Blend until uniform and smooth, for about 30 seconds.

3. Pour in smoothie glasses, add the ice cubes and sprinkle with cinnamon.

Nutrition for Total Servings:

Calories: 288

Fat: 6.4g

Carbs: 1 g

Protein: 1.4g

Raspberry Vanilla Shake

Preparation time: 5 minutes

Cooking time: 0 minutes

Servings: 2

Ingredients:

- 2 cups raspberries
- 2 tbsp. erythritol
- 6 raspberries to garnish
- 1/2 cup cold unsweetened soy milk
- 2/3 tsp. vanilla extract
- 1/2 cup heavy whipping cream

Directions:

1. In a large blender, process the raspberries, soy milk, vanilla extract, whipping cream, and erythritol for 2 minutes; work in two batches if needed.

2. The shake should be frosty.

3. Pour into glasses, stick in straws, garnish with raspberries, and serve.

Nutrition for Total Servings:

Calories: 298

Fat: 5.1g

Carbs: 1.2 g

Protein: 1.4g

COOKING CONVERSION CHART

Measurement				Temperature		Weight	

CUP	ONCES	MILLILITERS	TABLESPOONS	FAHRENHEIT	CELSIUS	IMPERIAL	METRIC
8 cup	64 oz	1895 ml	128	100 °F	37 °C	1/2 oz	15 g
6 cup	48 oz	1420 ml	96	150 °F	65 °C	1 oz	29 g
5 cup	40 oz	1180 ml	80	200 °F	93 °C	2 oz	57 g
4 cup	32 oz	960 ml	64	250 °F	121 °C	3 oz	85 g
2 cup	16 oz	480 ml	32	300 °F	150 °C	4 oz	113 g
1 cup	8 oz	240 ml	16	325 °F	160 °C	5 oz	141 g
3/4 cup	6 oz	177 ml	12	350 °F	180 °C	6 oz	170 g
2/3 cup	5 oz	158 ml	11	375 °F	190 °C	8 oz	227 g
1/2 cup	4 oz	118 ml	8	400 °F	200 °C	10 oz	283 g
3/8 cup	3 oz	90 ml	6	425 °F	220 °C	12 oz	340 g
1/3 cup	2.5 oz	79 ml	5.5	450 °F	230 °C	13 oz	369 g
1/4 cup	2 oz	59 ml	4	500 °F	260 °C	14 oz	397 g
1/8 cup	1 oz	30 ml	3	525 °F	274 °C	15 oz	425 g
1/16 cup	1/2 oz	15 ml	1	550 °F	288 °C	1 lb	453 g

Conclusion

Now that you are familiar with the Keto diet on many levels, you should feel confident in your ability to start your own Keto journey. This diet plan isn't going to hinder you or limit you, so do your best to keep this in mind as you begin changing your lifestyle and adjusting your eating habits. Packed with good fats and plenty of protein, your body is going to go through a transformation as it works to see these things as energy. Before you know it, your body will have an automatically accessible reserve that you can utilize at any time. Whether you need a boost of energy first thing in the morning or a second wind to keep you going throughout the day, this will already be inside of you.

As you take care of yourself through the afterward few years, you can feel great knowing that the Keto diet aligns with the anti-aging lifestyle you seek.

Not only does it keep you looking great and feeling younger, but it also acts as a preventative barrier from various ailments and conditions. The body tends to weaken as you age, but Keto helps keep a shield up in front of it by giving you plenty of opportunities to burn energy and create muscle mass.

Instead of taking the things you need to feel great, Keto only takes what you have in abundance. This is how you will always end up feeling your best each day.

Arguably one of the best diets around, Keto keeps you feeling great because you have many meal options! There is no shortage of delicious and filling meals you can eat while you are on any Keto diet plans. You can even take this diet with you as you eat out at restaurants and friends' houses. As long as you can remember the simple guidelines, you should have no problems staying on track with Keto. Cravings become almost non-existent as your body works to change the way it digests. Instead of relying on glucose in your bloodstream, your body switches focus. It begins using fat as soon as you reach the state of ketosis that you are aiming for. The best part is, you do not have to do anything other than eating within your fat/protein/carb percentages. Your body will do the rest on its own.

Because this is a way that your body can properly function for long periods, Keto is proven to be more than a simple fad diet. Originating with a medical background for helping epilepsy patients, the Keto diet has been tried and tested for decades. Many successful studies align with the knowledge that Keto works. Whether you are trying to be on a diet for a month or a year, both are just as healthy for you. Keto is an adjustment, but it will continue benefiting you for as long as you can keep it up. Good luck on your journey ahead!

CPSIA information can be obtained
at www.ICGtesting.com
Printed in the USA
BVHW091047090621
609091BV00008B/762